Intermittent

Fasting

Meal Plan

How to Make Your Life Healthier and Happier with Daily Meals Optimized for People on Intermittent Fasting

Estelle Chambers

TABLE OF CONTENTS

SMOOTHIES AND DRINKS..93

DESSERTS..97

INTRODUCTION

Intermittent fasting, also known as time-limited eating, is the practice of consuming food within a specific time frame or window. Basically, intermittent fasting consists of limiting food on the basis of specific times of day, days or days of the week.

Intermittent fasting gives you the advantage of being allowed to consume fewer calories over a longer period. The extended fasting period allows your body to stay in a fat and burn state longer than a daily or weekly interrupted fasting plan.

If you are considering trying intermittent fasting, here are a few types of intermittent fasting recipe plans you can follow. If you are already following the Keto diet, you will find that fasting windows and intermittent fasting plans can be managed just as well as a daily or weekly diet.

We have created some of the best Fast-Friendly Recipes that you can use according to your goals, from quick start to intermittent fasting, long term fasting and more. Each recipe has its own goals and benefits.

Read on to learn more about the different fasting periods you can follow, what foods and drinks you can eat and how to maximise the impact of intermittent fasting. As the name suggests, intermittent fasting is the practice of fasting with intermittent diets or not at all.

If you choose intermittent fasting, you should remember that your eating habits are not for everyone and you need to adjust your fasting plan. Your body will tell you that you need to eat a healthy diet, but your eating behavior is not like everyone else's. Although the intermittent fasting plan 16.8 does not specify which foods to eat and which to avoid, it is beneficial to focus on healthy eating to limit and avoid junk food.

Finally, it is helpful to understand that almost all of us follow intermittent fasting programs, even if they are not called "intermittent fasting." For many people, intermittent fasting is simply an eating behavior, and for most people, it means eating a few times a day. It is not a diet plan or exercise programme, but rather a way of controlling when and what you eat without focusing on diet. Before you start intermittent fasting, eat six or seven small meals a day and skip some meals consciously.

I usually follow the Leangain model of intermittent fasting, which uses a 16-hour fast followed by an 8-hour meal.

If you want to try intermittent fasting a legitimate method is to fast for 18 hours a day and eat every six hours, then give a month to see if it is right. If you fast for 18 hours a day, you will probably have to go through several months of fasting and eating.

If you are serious about results, you will find a way, after all, it is called intermittent fasting. Give intermittent fasting a chance, track your results and see how your body's blood formation changes as a result of this fast.

BREAKFAST RECIPES

1.Cheesy Chicken Cauliflower

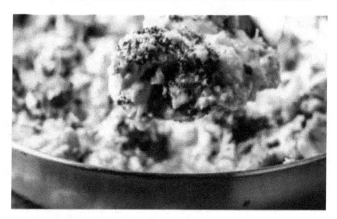

Preparation Time: 5 minutes

Cooking Time: 10 minutes

Servings: 4

Ingredients:

- 2 cups cauliflower florets, chopped
- ½ cup red bell pepper, chopped
- 1 cup roasted chicken, shredded (Lunch Recipes: Roasted Lemon Chicken Sandwich)
- ¼ cup shredded cheddar cheese
- 1 tablespoon. butter
- 1 tablespoon. sour cream
- Salt and pepper to taste

Directions:

1. Stir fry the cauliflower and peppers in the butter over medium heat until the veggies are tender.

2. Add the chicken and cook until the chicken is warmed through.

3. Add the remaining ingredients and stir until the cheese is melted.

4. Serve warm.

Nutrition: Calories: 144 kcal Carbs: 4 g Fat: 8.5 g Protein: 13.2 g.

2.Chicken Avocado Salad

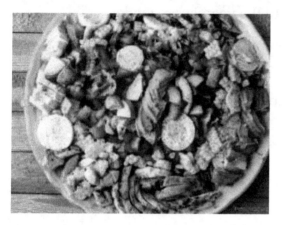

Preparation Time: 7 minutes

Cooking Time: 10 minutes

Servings: 4

Ingredients:

- 1 cup roasted chicken, shredded (Lunch Recipes: Roasted Lemon Chicken Sandwich)
- 1 bacon strip, cooked and chopped
- 1/2 medium avocado, chopped
- ¼ cup cheddar cheese, grated
- 1 hard-boiled egg, chopped
- 1 cup romaine lettuce, chopped
- 1 tablespoon. olive oil
- 1 tablespoon. apple cider vinegar
- Salt and pepper to taste

Directions:

1. Create the dressing by mixing apple cider vinegar, oil, salt and pepper.

2. Combine all the other ingredients in a mixing bowl.

3. Drizzle with the dressing and toss.

4. Can be refrigerated for up to 3 days.

Nutrition: Calories: 220 kcal Carbs: 2.8 g Fat: 16.7 g Protein: 14.8 g.

3.Chicken Broccoli Dinner

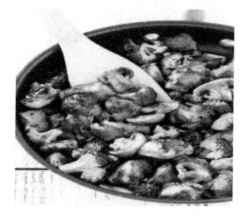

Preparation Time: 10 minutes

Cooking Time: 5 minutes

Servings: 1

Ingredients:

- 1 roasted chicken leg (Lunch Recipes: Roasted Lemon Chicken Sandwich)
- ½ cup broccoli florets
- ½ tablespoon. unsalted butter, softened
- 2 garlic cloves, minced
- Salt and pepper to taste

Directions:

1. Boil the broccoli in lightly salted water for 5 minutes. Drain the water from the pot and keep the broccoli in the pot. Keep the lid on to keep the broccoli warm.

2. Mix all the butter, garlic, salt and pepper in a small bowl to create garlic butter.

3. Place the chicken, broccoli and garlic butter.

Nutrition: Calories: 257 kcal Carbs: 5.1 g Fat: 14 gProtein: 27.4 g.

4.Easy Meatballs

Preparation Time: 10 minutes

Cooking Time: 20 minutes

Servings: 4

Ingredients:

- 1 lb. ground beef
- 1 egg, beaten
- Salt and pepper to taste
- 1 teaspoon garlic powder
- 1 teaspoon onion powder
- 2 tablespoons. butter
- ¼ cup mayonnaise
- ¼ cup pickled jalapeños
- 1 cup cheddar cheese, grated

Directions

1. Combine the cheese, mayonnaise, pickled jalapenos, salt, pepper, garlic powder and onion powder in a large mixing bowl.
2. Add the beef and egg and combine using clean hands.
3. Form large meatballs. Makes about 12.
4. Fry the meatballs in the butter over medium heat for about 4 minutes on each side or until golden brown.
5. Serve warm with a intermittent-friendly side.

6. The meatball mixture can also be used to make a meatloaf. Just preheat your oven to 400 degrees F, press the mixture into a loaf pan and bake for about 30 minutes or until the top is golden brown.

7. Can be refrigerated for up to 5 days or frozen for up to 3 months.

Nutrition: Calories: 454 kcal Carbs: 5 g Fat: 28.2 g Protein: 43.2 g.

5.Chicken Casserole

Preparation Time: 10 minutes

Cooking Time: 40 minutes

Servings: 8

Ingredients:

- 1 lb. boneless chicken breasts, cut into 1" cubes
- 2 tablespoons. butter
- 4 tablespoons. green pesto
- 1 cup heavy whipping cream
- ¼ cup green bell peppers, diced
- 1 cup feta cheese, diced
- 1 garlic clove, minced
- Salt and pepper to taste

Directions

1. Preheat your oven to 400 degrees F.
2. Season the chicken with salt and pepper then batch fry in the butter until golden brown.
3. Place the fried chicken pieces in a baking dish. Add the feta cheese, garlic and bell peppers.
4. Combine the pesto and heavy cream in a bowl. Pour on top of the chicken mixture and spread with a spatula.
5. Bake for 30 minutes or until the casserole is light brown around the edges.

6. Serve warm.

7. Can be refrigerated for up to 5 days and frozen for 2 weeks.

Nutrition: Calories: 294 kcal Carbs: 1.7 g Fat: 22.7 g Protein: 20.1 g.

6.Lemon Baked Salmon

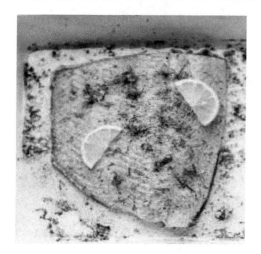

Preparation Time: 10 minutes

Cooking Time: 30 minutes

Servings: 4

Ingredients:

- 1 lb. salmon
- 1 tablespoon. olive oil
- Salt and pepper to taste
- 1 tablespoon. butter
- 1 lemon, thinly sliced
- 1 tablespoon. lemon juice

Directions:

1. Preheat your oven to 400 degrees F.
2. Grease a baking dish with the olive oil and place the salmon skin-side down.

3. Season the salmon with salt and pepper then top with the lemon slices.

4. Slice half the butter and place over the salmon.

5. Bake for 20minutes or until the salmon flakes easily.

6. Melt the remaining butter in a saucepan. When it starts to bubble, remove from heat and allow to cool before adding the lemon juice.

7. Drizzle the lemon butter over the salmon and Serve warm.

Nutrition: Calories: 211 kcal Carbs: 1.5 g Fat: 13.5 g Protein: 22.2 g.

LUNCH RECIPES

7.Thai Inspired Cashew Chicken

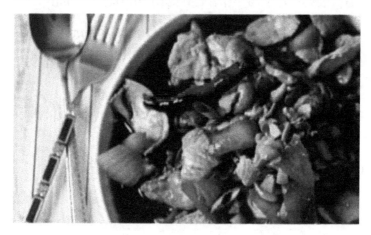

Preparation time: 5 minutes

Cooking time: 35 minutes

Servings: 4

Ingredients:

- 2 chicken breasts, cut into small pieces
- 2 chicken thighs, cut into small pieces
- 3 tablespoons coconut oil
- teaspoon ginger, minced
- teaspoon garlic, minced
- 1/2 medium green bell pepper, diced
- 1/4 cup raw cashews. Soaked for 30 minutes in water in refrigerated.
- small red onion, diced
- tablespoons soy sauce

- 1/2 tablespoon rice wine vinegar
- Salt
- Pepper

Directions:

1. In a pan, roast the cashews till browned. Set aside to cool.
2. Transfer to a food processor and grind. When the texture is grainy, add a little water and grind some more. Keep repeating until a paste is formed to your desired thickness.
3. Add the ginger, garlic, onion, bell pepper and oil to the pan and fry until the onions are golden brown.
4. Toss the chicken into the mix and cook on a medium heat.
5. Once cooked, add the salt, pepper, vinegar and soy sauce and reduce the mixture until the chicken is fully coated.
6. Enjoy.

Nutrition: Calorie count- 1267   Protein- 90g Carbs- 43g Fat- 104g

8.Garlic Butter Cod

Preparation time: 5 minutes

Cooking time: 20 minutes

Servings: 2

Ingredients:

- 3 cod fillets, 8 ounces each
- ¾ pound baby bok choy halved
- 1/3 cup butter, thinly sliced
- 1½ tablespoon garlic, minced
- Sea salt, as needed
- Freshly ground black pepper

Directions

1. Preheat your oven to 400 degrees Fahrenheit.
2. Cut 3 sheets of aluminum foil, large enough to accommodate one fillet.
3. Place cod fillets on each of the sheets and add butter and garlic on top of the fillets.
4. Add bok choy and season with pepper and salt according to your taste.
5. Fold the packet and enclose them in pouches.
6. Arrange on your baking sheet.
7. Bake for 20 minutes and transfer to a cooling rack.
8. Enjoy!

Nutrition: Calories: 355 Fat: 21g Net Carbohydrates: 3g Protein: 37g Fiber: 1g Carbohydrates: 5g

9.Broccoli & Tilapia

Preparation time: 4 minutes

Cooking time: 14 minutes

Servings: 2

Ingredients:

- 6 ounce of tilapia, frozen
- tablespoon butter
- tablespoon garlic, minced
- teaspoon lemon pepper seasoning
- cup broccoli florets, fresh

Directions:

1. Preheat your oven to 350 degrees Fahrenheit.
2. Add fish in aluminum foil packets.
3. Arrange broccoli around fish.
4. Sprinkle lemon pepper on top.
5. Close the packets and seal.
6. Bake for 14 minutes.
7. Take a bowl and add garlic and butter, mix well, and keep the mixture on the side.
8. Remove the packet from the oven and transfer it to a platter.
9. Place butter on top of the fish and broccoli, serve and enjoy!

Nutrition: Calories: 362 Fat: 25g Net Carbohydrates: 2g Protein: 29g Fiber: 1g Carbohydrates: 4g

10.Mexican Beef Zucchini Boats

Preparation time: 5 minutes

Cooking time: 20 minutes

Servings: 2

Ingredients:

- 1/2 pound ground beef
- tablespoon olive oil
- 1/2 teaspoon salt
- tablespoon Tex-Mex seasoning
- 1/2 teaspoon salt
- ½ cup fresh cilantro, finely chopped
- 1/2 tablespoon olive oil
- zucchini
- 1¼ cups cheese, grated
- ¼ cup black olives, sliced

Directions:

1. Preheat your oven to 400 degrees Fahrenheit. Split the zucchini in half lengthwise and remove the seed. Season with salt and let them sit for 10 minutes. Take a frying pan and place it over medium heat. Add olive oil and let the oil heat up. Season ground meat with salt and Tex-Mex seasoning. Pour meat to the frying pan. Cook until the liquid has evaporated. Blot off drops of liquid with a kitchen towel. Place zucchini halves in a greased baking dish. Mix 1/3rd of the cheese into ground beef alongside finely chopped cilantro, mix well. Divide the mixture between your zucchini boats.

Put olives on the top. Cover with grated cheese. Bake for 20 minutes. Let them cool for 5 minutes. Enjoy!

Nutrition: Calories: 60 Fat: 49g Net Carbohydrates: 6g Protein: 33g Fiber: 2g Carbohydrates: 8g

11. Avocado Beef Patties

Preparation time: 15 minutes

Cooking time: 10minutes

Servings: 2

Ingredients:

- pound 85% lean ground beef
- small avocado, pitted and peeled
- slices yellow cheddar cheese
- Salt, as needed
- Fresh ground black pepper, as needed

Directions:

1. Preheat and prepare your broiler to high. Divide beef into two equal-sized patties. Season the patties with salt and pepper accordingly. Broil the patties for 5 minutes per side. Place the patties on a platter and add cheese. Slice avocado into strips and place them on top of the patties. Serve and enjoy!

Nutrition: Calories: 568 Fat: 43g Net Carbohydrates: 9g Protein: 38g Fiber: 3g Carbohydrates: 12g

12.Chicken & Cabbage Platter

Preparation time: 9 minutes

Cooking time: 14 minutes

Servings: 2

Ingredients:

- ½ cup onion, sliced
- tablespoon sesame garlic-flavored oil
- cups Bok-Choy/Spinach, shredded
- 1/2 cup fresh bean sprouts
- 1½ stalks celery, chopped
- 1½ teaspoon garlic, minced
- 1/2 teaspoon stevia
- 1/2 cup chicken broth
- tablespoon coconut aminos
- 1/2 tablespoon freshly minced ginger 2 boneless chicken breast salt, to taste
- pepper, to taste

Directions:

1. Cut chicken breasts into pieces, season with salt and pepper. Fry it in the pan with garlic. Add chicken broth and sauté for a while.
2. Shred the cabbage with a knife.
3. Add onion, bean sprouts, celery, and sauté it until tender. Add stevia, coconut aminos, and ginger. Season with salt and pepper according to your taste.
4. Place the braised cabbage to your platter alongside the rotisserie chicken.

5. Enjoy!

Nutrition: Calories: 368 Fat: 18g Net Carbohydrates: 8g Protein: 42g Fiber: 3g Carbohydrates: 11g

13.Balsamic Chicken and Vegetables

Preparation time: 15 minutes

Cooking time: 10minutes

Servings: 4

Ingredients:

- 4 chicken thigh, boneless and skinless
- 5 stalks of asparagus, halved
- bell pepper, cut in chunks
- 1/2 red onion, diced
- garlic cloves, minced
- 2-ounces mushrooms, diced
- ¼ cup balsamic vinegar
- tablespoon olive oil
- ½ teaspoon stevia
- ½ tablespoon oregano
- Salt and pepper, as needed

Directions:

1. Preheat your oven to 425 degrees Fahrenheit. Mix the spices, olive oil, and vinegar. Combine the vegetables and mushrooms in a bowl.
2. Season with spices and sprinkle with oil.
3. Dip the chicken pieces into a spice mix and coat them thoroughly.
4. Place the veggies and chicken onto a pan in a single layer.
5. Cook for 25 minutes.
6. Serve and enjoy!

Nutrition: Calories: 401 Fat: 17g Net Carbohydrates: 11g Protein: 48g Fiber: 3g Carbohydrates: 14g

14. Onion Bacon Pork Chops

Preparation time: 10 minutes

Cooking time: 45 minutes

Servings: 2

Ingredients:

- onion, peeled and chopped
- bacon slices, chopped
- 1/4 cup chicken stock
- Salt and pepper to taste
- pork chops

Directions:

1. Heat a pan over medium heat and add bacon. Stir and cook until crispy. Transfer to a bowl. Return pan to medium heat and add onions, season with salt and pepper. Stir and cook for 15 minutes. Transfer to the same bowl with bacon. Return the pan to heat (medium-high) and add pork chops. Season with salt, pepper, and brown for 3 minutes. Flip and lower heat to medium. Cook for 7 minutes more. Add stock and stir cook for 2 minutes. Return the bacon and onions to the pan and stir cook for 1 minute. Serve and enjoy!

Nutrition: Calories: 325 Fat,: 18g Carbohydrates: 6g Protein: 36g Fiber: 2g Net Carbohydrates: 4g

15. Caramelized Pork Chops

Preparation time: 5 minutes

Cooking time: 30 minutes

Servings: 2

Ingredients:

- 2 pounds chuck roast, sliced
- 2 ounces green chili, chopped
- tablespoon chili powder
- 1/4 teaspoon dried oregano
- 1/4 teaspoon ground cumin
- garlic cloves, minced
- tablespoons olive oil
- Salt as needed

Directions:

1. Rub up your chop with 1 teaspoon of pepper and 2 teaspoons of seasoning salt. Take a skillet and heat some oil over medium heat. Brown your pork chops on each side. Add some water   and chili to the pan. Cover it up and lower down the heat, simmer it for about 20 minutes. Turn your chops over and add the rest of the pepper and salt. Cover it up, cook until the water evaporates, and the chili turns to tender.
2. Remove the chops from your pan and serve with some peppers on top.

Nutrition: Calories: 271 Fat,: 19g Carbohydrates: 4g Protein: 27g Fiber: 2g Net Carbohydrates: 2g

16.Chicken Bacon Quesadilla

Preparation time: 10 minutes

Cooking time: 35 minutes

Servings: 2

Ingredients:

- ¼ cup ranch dressing
- ½ cup cheddar cheese, shredded
- 20 slices bacon, center-cut
- 2 cups grilled chicken, sliced

Directions:

1. Re-heat your oven to 400 degrees F.
2. Line baking sheet using parchment paper.
3. Bake bacon slices for 30 minutes.
4. Lay grilled chicken over bacon square, drizzling ranch dressing on top.
5. Sprinkle cheddar cheese and top with another bacon square.
6. Bake for 5 minutes more.
7. Slice and serve. Enjoy!

Nutrition: Calories: 619 Fat,: 35g Carbohydrates: 2g Protein: 79g Fiber: 1g Net Carbohydrates: 1g

17.Asian Beef Steak

Preparation time: 10 minutes

Cooking time: 5 minutes

Servings: 2

Ingredients:

- 2 tablespoon sriracha sauce
- tablespoon garlic, minced
- tablespoon ginger, freshly grated
- yellow bell pepper, cut in strips
- red bell pepper, chopped in thin strips
- tablespoon sesame oil, garlic flavored
- tablespoon stevia
- ½ teaspoon curry powder
- ½ teaspoon of rice wine vinegar
- 8-ounce beef sirloin, cut into strips
- cups of baby spinach, stemmed
- ½ head of butter of lettuce, torn

Nutrition: Calories: 415 Fat,: 30g Carbohydrates: 4g Protein: 81g Fiber: 2g Net Carbohydrates: 2g

18.Sesame-Crusted Tuna with Green Beans

Preparation Time: 15 minutes

Cooking Time: 5 minutes

Servings: 4

Ingredients:

- ¼ cup white sesame seeds
- ¼ cup black sesame seeds
- 4 (6-ounce) ahi tuna steaks
- Salt and pepper
- tablespoon olive oil
- tablespoon coconut oil
- cups green beans

Directions:

1. In a shallow dish, mix the two kinds of sesame seeds.
2. Season the tuna with pepper and salt.
3. Dredge the tuna in a mixture of sesame seeds.
4. Heat up to high heat the olive oil in a skillet, then add the tuna.
5. Cook for 1 to 2 minutes until it turns seared, then sear on the other side.
6. Remove the tuna from the skillet, and let the tuna rest while using the coconut oil to heat the skillet.
7. Fry the green beans in the oil for 5 minutes then use sliced tuna to eat.

Nutrition: Calories: 420 Fats: 23 Protein: 7 Carbohydrates: 0

19.Rosemary Roasted Pork with Cauliflower

Preparation Time: 10 minutes

Cooking Time: 20 minutes

Servings: 4

Ingredients:

- ½ pounds boneless pork tenderloin
- tablespoon coconut oil
- tablespoon fresh chopped rosemary
- Salt and pepper
- tablespoon olive oil
- cups cauliflower florets

Directions:

1. Rub the coconut oil into the pork, then season with the rosemary, salt, and pepper.
2. Heat up the olive oil over medium to high heat in a large skillet.
3. Add the pork on each side and cook until browned for 2 to 3 minutes.
4. Sprinkle the cauliflower over the pork in the skillet.
5. Reduce heat to low, then cover the skillet and cook until the pork is cooked through for 8 to 10 minutes.
6. Slice the pork with cauliflower and eat.

Nutrition: Calories: 320 Fats: 37 Protein: 3 Carbohydrates: 1

20. Grilled Salmon and Zucchini with Mango Sauce

Preparation Time: 5 minutes

Cooking Time: 10 minutes

Servings: 4

Ingredients:

- 4 (6-ounce) boneless salmon fillets
- tablespoon olive oil
- Salt and pepper
- large zucchini, sliced in coins
- tablespoons fresh lemon juice
- ½ cup chopped mango
- ¼ cup fresh chopped cilantro
- teaspoon lemon zest
- ½ cup canned coconut milk

Directions:

1. Preheat a grill pan to heat, and sprinkle with cooking spray liberally.
2. Brush with olive oil to the salmon and season with salt and pepper.
3. Apply lemon juice to the zucchini, and season with salt and pepper.
4. Put the zucchini and salmon fillets on the grill pan.
5. Cook for 5 minutes then turn all over and cook for another 5 minutes.
6. Combine the remaining ingredients in a blender and combine to create a sauce.

7. Serve the side-drizzled salmon filets with mango sauce and zucchini.

Nutrition: Calories: 350 Fats: 23 Protein: 7 Carbohydrates: 6

21. Beef and Broccoli Stir-Fry

Preparation Time: 20 minutes

Cooking Time: 15 minutes

Servings: 4

Ingredients:

- ¼ cup soy sauce
- tablespoon sesame oil
- teaspoon garlic chili paste
- 1-pound beef sirloin
- tablespoons almond flour
- tablespoons coconut oil
- cups chopped broccoli florets
- tablespoon grated ginger
- cloves garlic, minced

Directions:

1. In a small bowl, whisk the soy sauce, sesame oil, and chili paste together.
2. In a plastic freezer bag, slice the beef and mix with the almond flour.
3. Pour in the sauce and toss to coat for 20 minutes, then let rest.
4. Heat up the oil over medium to high heat in a large skillet.
5. In the pan, add the beef and sauce and cook until the beef is browned.
6. Move the beef to the skillet sides, then add the broccoli, ginger, and garlic.

7. Sauté until tender-crisp broccoli, then throw it all together and serve hot.

Nutrition: Calories: 350 Fats: 19 Protein: 37 Carbohydrates: 6

22. Parmesan-Crusted Halibut with Asparagus

Preparation Time: 10 minutes

Cooking Time: 15 minutes

Servings: 4

Ingredients:

- 2 tablespoons olive oil
- ¼ cup butter, softened
- Salt and pepper
- ¼ cup grated Parmesan
- 1-pound asparagus, trimmed
- 2 tablespoons almond flour
- 4 (6-ounce) boneless halibut fillets
- teaspoon garlic powder

Directions:

1. Preheat the oven to 400 F and line a foil-based baking sheet.
2. Throw the asparagus in olive oil and scatter over the baking sheet.
3. In a blender, add the butter, Parmesan cheese, almond flour, garlic powder, salt and pepper, and mix until smooth.
4. Place the fillets with the asparagus on the baking sheet, and spoon the Parmesan over the eggs.
5. Bake for 10 to 12 minutes, then broil until browned for 2 to 3 minutes.

Nutrition: Calories: 415 Fats: 26 Protein: 42 Carbohydrates: 3

23. Hearty Beef and Bacon Casserole

Preparation time: 25 minutes

Cooking time: 30 minutes

Servings: 8

Ingredients:

- 8 slices uncooked bacon
- medium head cauliflower, chopped
- ¼ cup canned coconut milk
- Salt and pepper
- pounds ground beef (80% lean)
- 8 ounces mushrooms, sliced
- large yellow onion, chopped
- cloves garlic, minced

Direction:

1. Preheat to 375 F on the oven.
2. Cook the bacon in a skillet until its crispness, then drain and chop on paper towels.
3. Bring to boil a pot of salted water, then add the cauliflower.
4. Boil until tender for 6 to 8 minutes then drain and add the coconut milk to a food processor.
5. Mix until smooth, then sprinkle with salt and pepper.
6. Cook the beef until browned in a pan, then wash the fat away.
7. Remove the mushrooms, onion, and garlic, then move to a baking platter.

8. Place on top of the cauliflower mixture and bake for 30 minutes.
9. Broil for 5 minutes on high heat, then sprinkle with bacon to serve.

Nutrition: Calories: 410 Fats: 25 Protein: 37 Carbohydrates: 6

SIDES DISHES

24.Turnips Mash

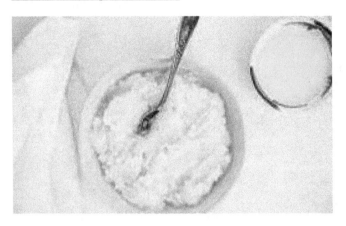

Preparation Time: 10 minutes

Cooking Time: 20 minutes

Servings: 4

Ingredients:

- 4 turnips, peeled and chopped
- ½ cup veggie stock
- Salt and black pepper to the taste
- yellow onion, chopped
- ¼ cup coconut cream

Directions:

1. In a pot, combine the turnips with stock and onion, stir, bring to a simmer, cook for 20 minutes and blend using an immersion blender.

2. Add salt, pepper and cream blend again, divide between plates and serve as a side dish.

Nutrition: Calories: 201 Fat: 3 Fiber: 3 Carbs: 7 Protein: 8

25.Cabbage Sauté

Preparation Time:5 minutes

Cooking Time: 10 minutes

Servings: 2

Ingredients:

- 3 ounces kale
- 2 ounces green cabbage
- 2 ounces red cabbage
- tablespoon lemon juice
- tablespoons olive oil
- ¼teaspoon black pepper
- Salt to taste

Directions:

1. Tear the kale leaves from stems, and cut the cabbage into thin pieces.
2. Take a skillet and heat the oil over a low to medium heat. Put everything into a skillet. Pour some lemon juice and season the mixture with some salt and pepper. Stir everything together.
3. Leave the skillet over medium heat and cook the mixture for 5-10 minutes or until you notice it became tender and golden at the edges.

Nutrition: Calories: 148 Total Carbs: 6g Fiber: 2g Net Carbs: 4g Fat: 14g Protein: 1,7g

26.Creamy Cabbage

Preparation Time: 5 minutes

Cooking Time: 10 minutes

Servings: 2

Ingredients:

- 6 ounces cabbage
- garlic clove
- tablespoon butter (or coconut oil)
- ounce vegetable broth (or water)
- ½ ounces heavy cream (or coconut cream)
- Salt to taste

Directions:

1. Cut the cabbage into thin slices and crush the garlic.
2. Take a large skillet and melt the butter over medium-high heat. Add in cabbage and garlic and cook for 3-4 minutes until you notice cabbage got tender.
3. Pour the broth and cream to the skillet and stir everything together. Wait until everything simmers and then cook it for 3-4 more minutes. You will know you are done when the cream is thick, and the cabbage is softer. Serve the meal while it's hot.

Nutrition: Calories: 149 Total Carbs: 6g Fiber: 1,6g Net Carbs: 4,4g Fat: 14,3g Protein: 1,9g

27. Creamy Coleslaw

Preparation Time: 10 minutes

Cooking Time: 2 minutes

Servings: 2

Ingredients:

- 3 ounces green cabbage
- ounce red cabbage
- ounces cucumber
- 6 black olives
- tablespoon scallions
- tablespoons mayonnaise
- ½ tablespoon lemon juice
- tablespoon dill
- tablespoon parsley
- Salt to taste

Directions:

1. Cut the red and green cabbage, olives, scallions, and cucumber into bite-sized pieces and add them to a bowl. Add some salt.
2. Put the lemon juice and mayo in another bowl. Mince the parsley and dill and combine them in.
3. Mix the wet and dry ingredients so you can prepare coleslaw. You can wait for the mixture to marinate a little bit and leave it aside for an hour or simply serve it right away

Nutrition: Calories: 222 Total Carbs: 6g Fiber: 2g Net Carbs: 4g Fat: 21g Protein: 1,5g

28.Crispy Bacon and Kale

Preparation Time: 5 minutes

Cooking Time: 14 minutes

Servings: 2

Ingredients:

- ½ ounces bacon
- 4 ounces kale
- ¼ teaspoon black pepper
- Salt to taste

Directions:

1. Take a wide pot (that will be suitable for kale you'll add later), and add bacon. Cook the strips over medium heat until they become crispy. Put them aside.
2. Lower the heat, cut your kale and place it in the pot. Cook the kale on the bacon grease for 5 minutes or until it becomes wilted. Toss in some pepper and salt.
3. Slice the bacon into smaller pieces and mix it with the kale. Serve it warm!

Nutrition: Calories: 116 Total Carbs: 3,7g Fiber: 1,2g Net Carbs: 2,5g Fat: 7,7g Protein: 8,3g

MEATS RECIPES

29.Intermittent Beef Liver with Asian Dip

Preparation Time: 10 minutes

Cooking Time: 15 minutes

Servings: 10

Ingredients:

- lb. beef liver, whole
- 1/4 cup tamari sauce
- cloves garlic
- tsp fresh ginger
- tsp sesame oil

Directions:

1. Spot the meat liver into a pot secured with water and heat to the point of boiling. Bubble for 2-3 minutes and afterward pour the water with the filth out. Top off with new water and bubble for 10 minutes.
2. In the interim, make the plunge by combining all the plunge ingredients.
3. Let the hamburger liver cool, at that point, cut it daintily and appreciate with the plunge.

Nutrition: Calories 66 Fat 2g Carbs 2g Protein 9g

30.Meatloaf Muffins

Preparation Time: 5 minutes

Cooking Time: 45 minutes

Servings: 6

Ingredients:

- pound ground beef
- cup chopped spinach
- large egg, lightly beaten
- ½ cup shredded mozzarella cheese
- ½ cup shredded parmesan cheese
- ¼ cup chopped yellow onion
- tbsp. seeded and minced jalapeno pepper

Directions:

1. Set the oven to 350F. Lightly grease every muffin tin.
2. Put and mix all ingredients in a bowl.
3. Scoop an equal portion of meat mixture into each muffin tin and press down lightly.
4. Bake for 45 minutes.
5. Serve.

Nutrition: Calories 198 Fat 13.8g Carbs 1.8g Protein 11.9g

31.Coffee Barbecue Pork Belly

Preparation Time: 15 minutes

Cooking Time: 60 minutes

Servings: 4

Ingredients:

- 1/2 cups beef stock
- pounds of pork belly
- tbsp. olive oil
- batch Low Carb Barbecue Dry Rub
- tbsp. Instant Espresso Powder

Directions:

1. Preheat the broiler to 350F.
2. Warmth the hamburger stock in a little pan over medium warmth until hot yet not bubbling
3. In a little bowl, combine the grill dry rub and coffee powder until very much joined.
4. Spot the pork midsection, skin side up in a shallow dish and sprinkle 2 tablespoons of the olive oil over the top, scouring it over the whole pork tummy.
5. Pour the hot stock around the pork midsection and spread the dish firmly with aluminum foil. Prepare for 45 minutes. Cut into 8 thick cuts.
6. Warmth the staying olive oil in a skillet over medium-high warmth and singe each cut for 3 minutes on each side or until the ideal degree of freshness is come to.

Nutrition: Calories 464 Fat 68g Carbs 3.4g Protein 24g

POULTRY

32.Parsnip & Bacon Chicken Bake

Preparation Time: 10 minutes

Cooking Time: 50 minutes

Servings: 4

Ingredients:

- 6 bacon slices, chopped
- 2 tbsp butter
- ½ lb. parsnips, diced
- 2 tbsp olive oil
- 1 lb. ground chicken
- 2 tbsp butter
- 1 cup heavy cream
- 2 oz. cream cheese, softened
- 1 ¼ cups grated Pepper Jack
- ¼ cup chopped scallions

Directions:

1. Preheat oven to 300 F. Put the bacon in a pot and fry it until brown and crispy, 6 minutes; set aside. Melt butter in a skillet and sauté parsnips until softened and lightly browned. Transfer to a greased baking sheet.

2. Heat olive oil in the same pan and cook the chicken until no longer pink, 8 minutes. Spoon onto a plate and set aside too.

3. Add heavy cream, cream cheese, and two-thirds of the Pepper Jack cheese to the pot. Melt the ingredients over medium heat, frequently stirring, 7 minutes.

4. Spread the parsnips on the baking dish, top with chicken, pour the heavy cream mixture over, and scatter bacon and scallions.

5. Sprinkle the remaining cheese on top and bake until the cheese melts and is golden, 30 minutes. Serve warm.

Nutrition: Cal 757 Net Carbs 5.5g Fat 66g Protein 29g

33. Chicken Bake with Onion & Parsnip

Preparation Time: 15 minutes

Cooking Time: 30 minutes

Servings:

Ingredients:

- 3 parsnips, sliced
- 1 onion, sliced
- 4 garlic cloves, crushed
- 2 tbsp olive oil
- 2 lb. chicken breasts
- ½ cup chicken broth
- ¼ cup white wine
- Salt and black pepper to taste

Directions:

1. Preheat oven to 360 F. Warm oil in a skillet over medium heat and brown chicken for a couple of minutes, and transfer to a baking dish.

2. Arrange the vegetables around the chicken and add in wine and chicken broth. Bake for 25 minutes, stirring once. Serve warm.

Nutrition: Cal 278 Net Carbs 5.1g Fat 8.7g Protein 35g

34.Cucumber-Turkey Canapes

Preparation Time: 10 minutes

Cooking Time: 5 minutes

Servings: 6

Ingredients:

- 2 cucumbers, sliced
- 2 cups dices leftover turkey
- ¼ jalapeño pepper, minced
- 1 tbsp Dijon mustard
- ¼ cup mayonnaise
- Salt and black pepper to taste

Directions:

1. Cut mid-level holes in cucumber slices with a knife and set aside.
2. Mix turkey, jalapeno pepper, mustard, mayonnaise, salt, and black pepper in a bowl.
3. Carefully fill cucumber holes with turkey mixture and serve.

Nutrition: Cal 170 Net Carbs 1.3g Fat 14g Protein 10g

SEAFOOD RECIPES

35.Tuna Salad Cucumber Boats

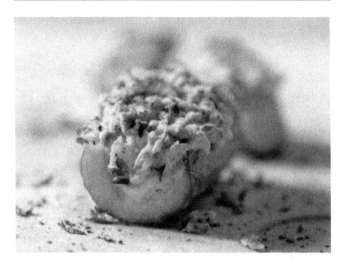

Preparation Time: 10 minutes

Cooking Time: 0 minutes;

Servings: 2

Ingredients

- 1 cucumber
- 2 oz. tuna, packed in water
- 1 green onion, sliced
- 2 1/2 tbsp. mayonnaise
- 1 tsp mustard paste
- Seasoning:
- ¼ tsp salt
- 1/8 tsp ground black pepper

Directions:

1. Prepare salad and for this, place tuna in a bowl, add onion, mayonnaise and mustard, then add salt and black pepper and stir until combined.
2. Cut cucumber from the middle lengthwise, then scrape out the inside by using a spoon and fill the space with tuna salad.
3. Serve.

Nutrition: 190 Calories; 14.2 g Fats; 8.8 g Protein; 3.6 g Net Carb; 2 g Fiber;

36.Salmon with Lime Butter Sauce

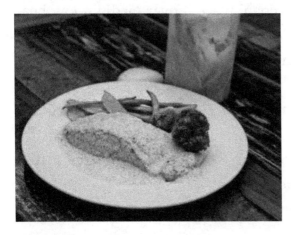

Preparation Time: 20 minutes

Cooking Time: 10 minutes;

Servings: 2

Ingredients

- 2 salmon fillets
- 1 lime, juiced, divided
- ½ tbsp. minced garlic
- 3 tbsp. butter, unsalted
- 1 tbsp. avocado oil
- Seasoning:
- 1/4 tsp salt
- 1/4 tsp ground black pepper

Directions:

1. Prepare the fillets and for this, season fillets with salt and black pepper, place them on a shallow dish, drizzle with half of the lime juice and then it marinate for 15 minutes.

2. Meanwhile, prepare the lime butter sauce and for this, take a small saucepan, place it over medium-low heat, add butter, garlic, and half of the lime juice, stir until mixed, and then bring it to a low boil, set aside until required.

3. Then take a medium skillet pan, place it over medium-high heat, add oil and when hot, place marinated salmon in it, cook for 3 minutes per side and then transfer to a plate.

4. Top each salmon with prepared lime butter sauce and then serve.

Nutrition: 192 Calories; 18 g Fats; 6 g Protein; 4 g Net Carb; 0 g Fiber;

37.Blackened Fish with Zucchini Noodles

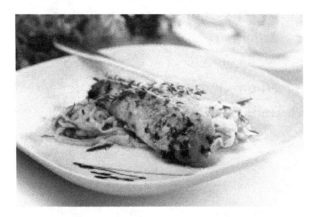

Preparation Time: 10 minutes;

Cooking Time: 12 minutes;

Servings: 2

Ingredients

- 1 large zucchini
- 2 fillets of mahi-mahi
- 1 tsp Cajun seasoning
- 2 tbsp. butter, unsalted
- 1 tbsp. avocado oil
- Seasoning:
- ½ tsp garlic powder
- 2/3 tsp salt
- ½ tsp ground black pepper

Directions:

1. Spiralized zucchini into noodles, place them into a colander, sprinkle with 1/3 tsp salt, toss until mixed and set aside until required.

2. Meanwhile, prepare fish and for this, season fillets with remaining salt and ¾ tsp Cajun seasoning.
3. Take a medium skillet pan, place it over medium heat, add butter and when it melts, add prepared fillets, switch heat to medium-high level and cook for 3 to 4 minutes per side until cooked and nicely browned.
4. Transfer fillets to a plate and then reserve the pan for zucchini noodles.
5. Squeeze moisture from the noodles, add them to the skillet pan, add oil, toss until mixed, season with remaining Cajun seasoning and cook for 2 to 3 minutes until noodles have turned soft.
6. Sprinkle with garlic powder, remove the pan from heat and distribute noodles between two plates.
7. Top noodles with a fillet and then serve.

Nutrition: 350 Calories; 25 g Fats; 27.1 g Protein; 2.8 g Net Carb; 1.6 g Fiber;

38.Garlic Parmesan Mahi-Mahi

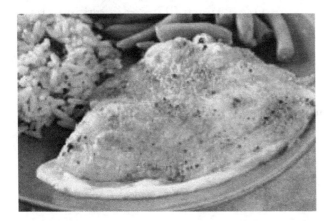

Preparation Time: 10 minutes

Cooking Time: 10 minutes;

Servings: 2

Ingredients

- 2 fillets of mahi-mahi
- 1 tsp minced garlic
- 1/3 tsp dried thyme
- 1 tbsp. avocado oil
- 1 tbsp. grated parmesan cheese
- Seasoning:
- 1/3 tsp salt
- 1/4 tsp ground black pepper

Directions:

1. Turn on the oven, set it to 425 degrees F and let it preheat.
2. Meanwhile, take a small bowl, place oil in it, add garlic, thyme, cheese and oil and stir until mixed.

3. Season fillets with salt and black pepper, then coat with prepared cheese mixture, place fillets in a baking sheet and then cook for 7 to 10 minutes until thoroughly cooked.

4. Serve.

Nutrition: 170 Calories; 7.8 g Fats; 22.3 g Protein; 0.8 g Net Carb; 0 g Fiber;

VEGETABLES

39.African Sweet Potato Stew

Preparation Time: 15 Minutes

Cooking Time: 7 To 8 Hours

Servings: 4

Ingredients:

- 4 cups peeled diced sweet potatoes
- 1 (15-ounce) can red kidney beans, drained and rinsed
- 1 (14.5-ounce) can diced tomatoes, drained
- 1 cup diced red bell pepper
- 2 cups Very Easy Vegetable Broth (here) or store bought
- 1 medium yellow onion, chopped
- 1 (4.5-ounce) can chopped green chilis, drained
- 1 teaspoon minced garlic (2 cloves)
- 1½ teaspoons ground ginger
- 1 teaspoon ground cumin
- 4 tablespoons creamy peanut butter
- Pinch salt
- Freshly ground black pepper

Directions:

1. Combine the sweet potatoes, kidney beans, diced tomatoes, bell pepper, vegetable broth, onion, green chilis, garlic, ginger, and cumin in a slow cooker. Mix well

2. Cover and cook on low for 7 to 8 hours.

3. Ladle a little of the soup into a small bowl and mix in the peanut butter, then pour the mixture back into the stew

4. Season with salt and pepper. Mix well and serve.

Nutrition: Calories: 514 Total fat: 10g Protein: 22g Sodium: 649mg Fiber: 17g

40.Jackfruit Cochinita Pibil

Preparation Time: 15 Minutes

Cooking Time: 8 Hours

Servings: 4

Ingredients:

- 2 (20-ounce) cans jackfruit, drained, hard pieces discarded
- 2/3 cup freshly squeezed lemon juice
- 1/3 cup orange juice
- 2 habanero peppers, seeded and chopped
- 2 tablespoons achiote paste
- 2 teaspoons ground cumin
- 2 teaspoons smoked paprika
- 2 teaspoons chili powder
- 2 teaspoons ground coriander
- Pinch salt
- Freshly ground black pepper
- Warmed corn tortillas, for serving

Directions:

1. Combine the jackfruit, lemon juice, orange juice, habanero peppers, achiote paste, cumin, smoked paprika, chili powder, and coriander in a slow cooker; mix well.

2. Cover and cook on low for 8 hours or on high for 4 hours.

3. Use two forks to pull the jackfruit apart into shreds. Season with salt and pepper.

4. Heat tortillas directly over a gas fire, or in a skillet over medium heat for about 1 minute per side. Spoon the jackfruit into the tortillas and serve.

Nutrition: Calories: 297 Total fat: 2g Protein: 5g Sodium: 71mg Fiber: 6g

41.Delightful Dal

Preparation Time: 15 Minutes

Cooking Time: 7 To 9 Hours

Servings: 4

Ingredients:

- 3 cups red lentils, rinsed
- 6 cups water
- 1 (28-ounce) can diced tomatoes, with juice
- 1 small yellow onion, diced
- 2½ teaspoons minced garlic (5 cloves)
- 1 (1-inch) piece fresh ginger, peeled and minced
- 1 tablespoon ground turmeric
- 2 teaspoons ground cumin
- 1½ teaspoons ground cardamom
- 1½ teaspoons whole mustard seeds
- 1 teaspoon fennel seeds
- 1 bay leaf
- 1 teaspoon salt
- ¼ teaspoon freshly ground black pepper

Directions:

1. Combine the lentils, water, diced tomatoes, onion, garlic, ginger, turmeric, cumin, cardamom, mustard

seeds, fennel seeds, bay leaf, salt, and pepper in a slow cooker; mix well.

2. Cover and cook on low for 7 to 9 hours or on high for 4 to 6 hours.

3. Remove the bay leaf, and serve.

Nutrition: Calories: 585 Total fat: 4g Protein: 40g Sodium: 616mg Fiber: 48g

42.Moroccan Chickpea Stew

Preparation Time: 15 Minutes

Cooking Time: 6 To 8 Hours

Servings: 4

Ingredients:

- 1 small butternut squash, peeled and chopped into bite-size pieces
- 3 cups Very Easy Vegetable Broth (here) or store bought
- 1 medium yellow onion, diced
- 1 bell pepper, diced
- 1 (15-ounce) can chickpeas, drained and rinsed
- 1 (14.5-ounce) can tomato sauce
- ¾ cup brown lentils, rinsed
- 1½ teaspoons minced garlic (3 cloves)
- 1½ teaspoons ground ginger
- 1½ teaspoons ground turmeric
- 1½ teaspoons ground cumin
- 1 teaspoon ground cinnamon
- ¾ teaspoon smoked paprika
- ½ teaspoon salt
- 1 (8-ounce) package fresh udon noodles
- Freshly ground black pepper

Directions:

1. Combine the butternut squash, vegetable broth, onion, bell pepper, chickpeas, tomato sauce, brown lentils, garlic, ginger, turmeric, cumin, cinnamon, smoked paprika, and salt in a slow cooker. Mix well.

2. Cover and cook 6 to 8 hours on low or 3 to 4 hours on high. In the last 10 minutes of cooking, add the noodles.

3. Season with pepper, and serve.

Nutrition: Calories: 427 Total fat: 4g Protein: 26g Sodium: 1,423mg Fiber: 24g

43.Broccoli Quinoa Casserole

Preparation Time: 15 minutes

Cooking Time: 30 minutes

Servings: 5

Ingredients:

- Four and a half cups of vegetable stock
- Two and a half cups of quinoa (uncooked)
- Half a tsp. of salt
- Two tablespoons of pesto sauce
- Two teaspoons of cornstarch
- Twelve ounces of mozzarella cheese (skimmed)
- Two cups of spinach (fresh and organic)
- One-third cup of parmesan cheese
- Three medium-sized green onions (chopped)
- Twelve ounces of broccoli florets (fresh)

Directions:

1. Set the temperature of the oven to 400 degrees Fahrenheit and preheat. Take a rectangular baking dish and add the quinoa to it along with the green onions. In the meantime, take a large-sized bowl and add the broccoli florets to it. Microwave the florets at high for about five minutes. Once done, set them aside.

2. Take a large-sized mixing bowl and in it, add the pesto, vegetable sauce, cornstarch, and salt. Use a wire whisk

to mix all of them properly. Now, heat this mixture until it starts to boil. You can either do this in the microwave, or you can use your stovetop as well.

3. Now, take the vegetable stock and the spinach and add them to the quinoa. Add the three-quarter of the mozzarella cheese and the parmesan as well. Bake the mixture for thirty to thirty-five minutes. Once done, take the casserole of quinoa out and then mix the broccoli into it. Take the rest of the cheese and sprinkle on top. Place the preparation back in the oven for another five minutes. By this time, all the cheese will melt.

Nutrition: Calories: 49 Protein: 27.6g Fat: 16g Carbs: 61.3g Fiber: 9g

SOUPS AND STEWS

44.Flu Soup

Preparation Time: 10 minutes

Cooking Time: 15 minutes

Servings: 4 servings

Ingredients:

- 1 cup mushrooms, chopped
- 1 cup spinach, chopped
- 3 oz. scallions, diced
- 2 oz. Cheddar cheese, shredded
- 1 teaspoon cayenne pepper
- 1 cup organic almond milk
- 2 cups chicken broth
- ½ teaspoon salt

Directions:

1. Put all Ingredients in the instant pot and close the lid.
2. Set the manual mode (high pressure) and cook the soup for 15 minutes.
3. Make a quick pressure release.
4. Blend the soup with the help of the immersion blender.
5. When the soup will get smooth texture – it is cooked.

Nutrition: Calories 228 Fat 19.9 Fiber 2.3 Carbs 6.6 Protein 8.5

45.Jalapeno Soup

Preparation Time: 10 minutes

Cooking Time: 10 minutes

Servings: 4 servings

Ingredients:

- 2 jalapeno peppers, sliced
- 3 oz. pancetta, chopped
- ½ cup heavy cream
- 2 cups of water
- ½ cup Monterey jack cheese, shredded
- ½ teaspoon garlic powder
- 1 teaspoon coconut oil
- ½ teaspoon smoked paprika

Directions:

1. Toss pancetta in the instant pot, add coconut oil and cook it for 4 minutes on sauté mode. Stir it from time to time.
2. After this, add sliced jalapenos, garlic powder, and smoked paprika.
3. Stir the Ingredients for 1 minute.
4. Add heavy cream and water.
5. Then add Monterey Jack cheese and stir the soup well.
6. Close and seal the lid; cook the soup for 5 minutes on manual mode (high pressure); make a quick pressure release.

Nutrition: Calories 234 Fat 20 Fiber 0.4 Carbs 1.7 Protein 11.8

46. Garden Soup

Preparation Time: 20 minutes

Cooking Time: 29 minutes

Servings: 5 servings

Ingredients:

- ½ cup cauliflower florets
- 1 cup kale, chopped
- 1 garlic clove, diced
- 1 tablespoon olive oil
- 1 teaspoon sea salt
- 6 cups beef broth
- 2 tablespoons chives, chopped

Directions:

1. Heat up olive oil in the instant pot on sauté mode for 2 minutes and add clove.
2. Cook the vegetables for 2 minutes and stir well.
3. Add kale, cauliflower, and sea salt, chives, and beef broth.
4. Close and seal the lid.
5. Cook the soup on manual mode (high pressure) for 5 minutes.
6. Then make a quick pressure release and open the lid.
7. Ladle the soup into the bowls.

Nutrition: Calories 80 Fat 4.5 Fiber 0.5 Carbs 2.3 Protein 6.5

47.Shirataki Noodle Soup

Preparation Time: 25 minutes

Cooking Time: 15 minutes

Servings: 2 servings

Ingredients:

- 2 oz. shirataki noodles
- 2 cups of water
- 6 oz. chicken fillet, chopped
- 1 teaspoon salt
- 1 tablespoon coconut aminos

Directions:

1. Pour water in the instant pot bowl.
2. Add salt and chopped chicken fillet. Close and seal the lid.
3. Cook the Ingredients on manual mode (high pressure) for 15 minutes. Allow the natural pressure release for 10 minutes.
4. After this, add shirataki noodles and coconut aminos.
5. Leave the soup for 10 minutes to rest.

Nutrition: Calories 175 Fat 6.3 Fiber 3 Carbs 1.5 Protein 24.8

48. Cordon Blue Soup

Preparation Time: 15 minutes

Cooking Time: 6 minutes

Servings: 4 servings

Ingredients:

- 4 cups chicken broth
- 7 oz. ham, chopped
- 3 oz. Mozzarella cheese, shredded
- 1 teaspoon ground black pepper
- ½ teaspoon salt
- 2 tablespoons ricotta cheese
- 2 oz. scallions, chopped

Directions:

1. Put all Ingredients in the instant pot bowl and stir gently.
2. Close and seal the lid; cook the soup on manual mode (high pressure) for 6 minutes.
3. Then allow the natural pressure release for 10 minutes and ladle the soup into the bowls.

Nutrition: Calories 196 Fat 10.1 Fiber 1.2 Carbs 5.3 Protein 20.3

49.Bacon Soup

Preparation Time: 10 minutes

Cooking Time: 20 minutes

Servings: 4 servings

Ingredients:

- 3 oz. bacon, chopped
- 1 cup cheddar cheese, shredded
- 1 tablespoon scallions, chopped
- 3 cups beef broth 1 cup of coconut milk
- 1 teaspoon curry powder

Directions:

1. Heat up the instant pot on sauté mode for 3 minutes and add bacon.
2. Cook it for 5 minutes. Stir it from time to time.
3. Then add scallions and curry powder. Cook the Ingredients for 5 minutes more. Stir them from time to time.
4. After this, add coconut milk and beef broth.
5. Add cheddar cheese and stir the soup well.
6. Cook it on manual mode (high pressure) for 10 minutes. Make a quick pressure release.
7. Mix up the soup well before serving.

Nutrition: calories 398 fat 33.6 fiber 1.5 carbs 5.1 protein 20

SNACKS

50. Cinnamon Butter

Preparation Time: 10 minutes + 1hour chilling

Cooking Time: 0 minutes

Servings: 8

Ingredients:

- ½ cup butter, at room temperature
- 5 drops liquid stevia
- ½ tsp. Pure vanilla extract
- ½ tsp. ground cinnamon
- 1/8 tsp. sea salt

Directions:

1. Combine the butter, vanilla, cinnamon, salt, and stevia in a large bowl. Mix well until smooth.
2. Line a baking sheet using a wax paper then spread the cinnamon butter mixture on top. Roll the paper to seal the butter mixture, then seal the ends.
3. Refrigerate the butter for 1 hour before using it. Store in the refrigerator for up to 2 weeks. Best served on the Intermittent Bread or with celery sticks.

Nutrition: Calories: 103 Fat: 12g Carbs: 0.1g Protein: 0.1g

51.Intermittent Bacon Burger Bombs

Preparation Time: 10 minutes

Cooking Time: 60 minutes

Servings: 12

Ingredients:

- 12 slices bacon
- 12 cubes smoked cheddar cheese, (1-inch)
- 12 rounds sausage patties, raw, (1-ounce)
- To taste: cumin, onion powder, salt, pepper

Directions:

1. Preheat oven to 350°F. Layout sausage rounds on a cookie sheet lined with parchment paper.
2. Dust sausage with cumin, onion powder, salt, and pepper.
3. Place a piece of cheese in the middle of the sausage rounds.
4. Form a ball around the cheese with the sausage. Roll it in your hands to make a good circle shape.
5. Wrap bacon around the sausage balls.
6. Bake at 350°F for an hour.
7. Enjoy with your favorite burger condiments!

Nutrition: Calories: 249 Fat: 20.4g Carbs: 1.3g Protein: 14.4g

52.Bacon Wrapped Chicken Bombs

Preparation Time: 15 minutes

Cooking Time: 35-45 minutes

Servings: 6

Ingredients:

- 2 lb. (about 3) boneless, skinless, chicken breasts
- 10 oz. frozen spinach
- 4 oz. cream cheese, softened
- ½ cup full-fat ricotta
- Salt and pepper to taste
- 12 slices bacon

Directions:

1. Thaw the spinach out, then wring with water.
2. Set the oven to 375°F.
3. Mix the spinach in the cream cheese and ricotta.
4. Season with salt and pepper to taste.
5. Chop the chicken breasts in half, as shown. You want them to be still thick enough to cut pouches into.
6. Cut pockets into 1 of the ends of every piece of chicken. Stuff the pockets with the cheese filling.
7. Wrap 2 slices of bacon around per piece of chicken. Seal the open end and any holes where filling might seep out.
8. Pan sear the bacon-wrapped chicken in a hot skillet. You do not have to brown all the sides equally because they will be finished off in the oven.

9. Set the pieces of chicken into an oven-safe dish while you finish the others.
10. Bake for at least 35-45 minutes until the bacon is well crisped, and the chicken is cooked all the way through. The chicken is completely cooked when it reaches 165°F.

Nutrition: Calories: 384.8 Fat: 20.5g Carbs: 2.3g Protein: 44.8g

SMOOTHIES AND DRINKS

53.Cinnamon Pear Protein Shake (soy, nuts)

Preparation Time: 5 minutes

Cooking Time: 0 minutes

Servings: 1

Ingredients:

- 1 tsp. freeze-dried pear powder
- 1 medium Hass avocado (peeled, pitted, and halved)
- 2 cups unsweetened almond milk
- 1 scoop organic soy protein (vanilla flavor)
- ½ tsp. cinnamon
- 4-6 drops stevia sweetener
- 2 ice cubes

Directions:

1. Add all the required ingredients to a blender, including the optional ice cubes if desired, and blend for 1 minute.

2. Transfer to a large cup or shaker and enjoy!

3. Alternatively, store the smoothie in an airtight container or a mason jar, keep it in the fridge, and

consume within 3 days. Store for a maximum of 30 days in the freezer and thaw at room temperature.

Nutrition: Calories: 398 kcal Net Carbs: 5.4 g. Fat: 28 g. Protein: 28.8 g. Fiber: 14.9 g. Sugar: 4.4 g.

54. Raspberry Coco Shake (soy, nuts)

Preparation Time: 5 minutes

Cooking Time: 0 minutes

Servings: 2

Ingredients:

- 1 ½ cups unsweetened almond milk
- 1 scoop organic soy protein (chocolate flavor)
- ½ cup full-fat coconut milk
- ½ cup raspberries (fresh or frozen)
- 4 drops stevia sweetener
- 2 ice cubes

Directions:

1. Put all the ingredients in a blender and blend for about 1 minute, or until the shake reaches the desired consistency.

2. Transfer the shake to a large cup or shaker and enjoy!

3. Alternatively, store the smoothie in an airtight container or mason jar in the fridge, and consume within 3 days. Store for a maximum of 30 days in the freezer and thaw at room temperature before serving.

Nutrition: Calories: 383 kcal Net Carbs: 5.6 g. Fat: 28.6 g. Protein: 24.6 g. Fiber: 6.5 g. Sugar: 4.8 g.

DESSERTS

55.Intermittent Cream Cheese Frosted Carrot Mug Cake

Preparation Time: 10 minutes

Cooking Time: 2 minutes

Servings: 2

Ingredients:

- Cake:
- 2 tablespoons almond flour
- tablespoon erythritol
- tablespoon psyllium husk
- tablespoon butter (melted)
- piece large egg (beaten lightly)
- teaspoon cinnamon
- 1/2 teaspoon vanilla extract
- 1/2 teaspoon baking powder
- 1/2 piece small carrot (grated finely)
- 1/4 teaspoon ginger (ground)
- pinch of salt
- Frosting:
- tablespoon whipping cream
- 1/4 cup cream cheese (room temperature)
- 1/2 teaspoon vanilla extract
- 1/2 tablespoon erythritol

Directions:

1. In a food processor, put in all the ingredients for the cake. Blend to combine everything.
2. Pour the blended mixture from the food processor into a microwave-safe mug.
3. Microwave it for 90 seconds on high setting.
4. Remove the cake from the mug. Set it aside to cool down.
5. Cut the cake into two layers. Set aside.
6. In a mixing bowl, put in the cream cheese, vanilla extract, and erythritol. Whip them up using an electric hand mixer. Continue whipping until the texture of the mixture becomes soft and creamy.
7. Put in the whipping cream into the cream cheese mixture. Mix thoroughly for 5 minutes.
8. Get the bottom layer of the cake. Scoop a heaping tablespoon of the cream cheese frosting. Spread the frosting on top of the bottom layer of the cake.
9. Get the top layer of the cake. Gently put it on top of the frosted bottom layer of the cake.
10. Spread the rest of the cream cheese frosting on top of the cake and on the sides.
11. You can chill the cake before serving, or you can serve it right away. Cut the cake in half and enjoy.

Nutrition: Calories: 229 Carbs: 20 g Fats: 17.3 g Proteins: 6 g Fiber: 15.9 g

56.Intermittent Avocado Brownies

Preparation Time: 10 minutes

Cooking Time: 30 minutes

Servings: 12

Ingredients:

- 2 pieces large avocadoes (ripe)
- 100 grams Lily's chocolate chips (melted)
- 4 tablespoons cocoa powder
- 3 tablespoons refined coconut oil
- 1/2 teaspoon vanilla
- 2 pieces eggs
- Dry Ingredients:
- 90 grams almond flour (blanched)
- 1/4 cup erythritol
- teaspoon baking powder
- teaspoon stevia powder
- 1/4 teaspoon baking soda
- 1/4 teaspoon salt

Directions:

1. Preheat your oven to 350 degrees Fahrenheit.
2. In a mixing bowl, put in all the ingredients listed under dry ingredients. Whisk to combine well. Set aside.
3. Cut the avocadoes in half. Scoop out the flesh. Weigh the avocadoes. You will need a total of 250 grams of avocadoes for this recipe.
4. Put the avocadoes in a food processor. Process the avocadoes until the texture becomes smooth.

5. Put in the rest of the ingredients into the food processor one at a time. Process for a few seconds after each ingredient is added into the avocado mixture.
6. Put in the flour mixture into the food processor. Process until everything is well combined.
7. Line a baking dish (12" x 8") with parchment paper. Transfer the avocado batter into the baking dish. Spread the batter evenly on the surface of the baking dish.
8. Bake the batter for 30 minutes. Do the toothpick test to know if the brownie is done. The top surface of the brownie should be soft to the touch.
9. Take the brownie out from the oven. Set it aside to cool down. Cut the brownie into 12 square pieces.

Nutrition: Calories: 155 Carbs: 9.78 g Fats: 14.05 g Proteins: 4.02 g Fiber: 6.98 g

CPSIA information can be obtained
at www.ICGtesting.com
Printed in the USA
LVHW082033040521
686473LV00008B/261